I0113860

THE

POLYVAGAL

THEORY

NEUROPHYSIOLOGICAL FOUNDATIONS OF COMMUNICATION, EMOTIONS, AND SELF-REGULATION - HARNESSING VAGUS NERVE'S HEALING POWER FOR TRAUMA, ANXIETY, CHRONIC ILLNESS & MENTAL STRESS.

YUMI PARK

Copyright © 2023 by Yumi Park

All rights reserved.

It is not legal to reproduce, duplicate, or transmit any part of this document in either electronic means or in printed format. Recording of this publication is strictly prohibited and any storage of this document is not allowed unless with written permission from the publisher except for the use of brief quotations in a book review.

ISBN: 9781835122969

CONTENTS

INTRODUCTION

Life often places us on a rollercoaster of emotional experiences, from moments of happiness and calm to periods of nervous tension. We might wonder how our bodies mostly navigate these ever-changing states with seeming agility. The answer lies within us, particularly within a unique theory centered around one cranial nerve—the tenth cranial nerve, also known as the vagus nerve. Welcome to the fascinating world of Polyvagal Theory.

When I met John, he was a senior manager at a multinational corporation, which I consulted during a particularly difficult time in social and economic environments worldwide. John seemed stressed and was struggling with emotional and mental balance.

One day, he shared with me that most of his relationships at work and home often broke down after a short while. When I asked why he thought that happened, he was quiet for a while, then acknowledged that he was not always feeling safe and secure, that he wanted to make the right decisions, and that always wanted to be liked. He was second-guessing himself, fluctuating between feeling frustrated, angry, withdrawn, and isolated. The few people whom he felt comfortable asking indicated that this seeming instability lessened their trust in him and made them cautious and wary.

Feeling his fear in my own autonomic nervous system, I recognized that he was probably poorly regulated. Despite the many reasons that could be at play from his past, I suggested that he read about polyvagal theory and applied some of the exercises experts recommend.

I thought about John occasionally over the course of many years until we met again at a conference. He was a totally different person from before. He told me that knowing about and applying the polyvagal theory completely changed his life.

So, before we catch up again with John, let us explore what Polyvagal Theory is all about.

1

THE BASICS OF THE POLYVAGAL THEORY

Introduction To The Polyvagal Theory

D eveloped by Dr. Stephen Porges in the 1990s , the Polyvagal Theory presents a revolutionary perspective on the way our nervous system interacts with our experiences. This theory centers around the functioning of the vagus nerve, one of the longest nerves in our body, and its crucial role in dictating our emotional and social behavior. By decoding the language of our nervous system, the Polyvagal Theory opens up new dimensions of understanding our physiological responses to safety and danger.

So, why does this matter? Well, the Polyvagal Theory is not just an academic topic for psychologists and neuroscientists. It is a concept that resonates with every breath we take, every emotion we feel, and every interaction we have. It is a hidden but substantial thread weaving through the fabric of our everyday experiences, connecting our internal bodily functions with our external social interactions while greatly affecting our mindset and mental wellbeing.

At the heart of the Polyvagal Theory lies a simple yet profound message: the state of our nervous system influences how we show up in the world. Our body's perception of safety or threat influences our ability to connect with others, express ourselves, function, and even love. The theory provides a physiological context to explain why we might feel socially connected and safe in some situations, while in others, we may experience fear, disconnect, and an intense urge to withdraw.

Understanding the Polyvagal Theory is like being handed a roadmap of our inner physiological landscape. It equips us with a new language to interpret our bodily signals and emotional states. By bringing into our conscious awareness the subconscious workings of our nervous system, the theory empowers us to be active participants in shaping our wellbeing. We eliminate blind spots about ourselves and others, and regulate ourselves better.

In the coming sections, we delve deeper into the evolution of the Polyvagal Theory, its principles, and its intricate relationship with the Autonomic Nervous System. As we unpack these concepts, keep in mind that this theory is not a distant scientific hypothesis, but our life story that plays out within us every day, influencing our life and relationships in more ways than we might realize.

This journey through the Polyvagal Theory is a discovery of the hidden dynamics of our being. It is about uncovering a new layer of self-awareness and embracing a fresh perspective on what it means to be human and resonate positively with other beings.

The Evolution Of Polyvagal Theory

Unraveling the threads of the Polyvagal Theory takes us back to the groundbreaking work of Dr. Stephen Porges in the late

20th century. Trained as a psychologist with a keen interest in the interplay of mind and body, Porges sought to understand the underlying physiology of our emotional experiences and automatic responses. His curiosity and exploration culminated in a pioneering neurophysiological theory that has revolutionized our understanding of human behavior and emotion—the Polyvagal Theory.

Before the advent of the Polyvagal Theory, the study of the autonomic nervous system was generally confined within a dichotomous framework, dividing our physiological responses into two states, namely fight-or-flight (sympathetic arousal) and rest-and-digest (parasympathetic calm). This binary model, however, left several physiological phenomena unexplained, stimulating Porges's curiosity to explore further.

Porges's journey into the unknown was fueled by a simple yet profound question: What if there is more to the human nervous system than just a binary toggle between arousal and calm? His pursuit of this question led to the formulation of the Polyvagal Theory, which uncovered a third type of autonomic response characterized by the type and intensity of social communication and connection.

Central to the Polyvagal Theory is the role of the vagus nerve. This tenth cranial nerve had been recognized by researchers for its involvement in parasympathetic activities such as rest and relax. However, Porges identified that the vagus nerve is not a single, unified entity. Instead, it comprises two distinct branches, each with different evolutionary origins and functions, leading to the prefix 'poly,' meaning 'many'.

Porges's work illuminated that the older, unmyelinated (i.e., lacking a myelinated or insulating sheath) branch of the vagus nerve, termed 'Dorsal Vagal,' is associated with immobilization behaviors, like fainting and freezing. On the other hand, the newer, myelinated branch, referred to as 'Ventral Vagal,' is linked to social engagement behaviors and the state of calm and relaxation. The dorsal nervous system comprises the spinal column, brain, spinal cord, and tissue surrounding these. The ventral nervous system is made up of the thoracic, abdominal, and pelvic cavities.

But the Polyvagal Theory's contribution extends beyond just scientific understanding—it offers a compassionate perspective towards our emotional responses. By providing a biological explanation for our reactions to stress and trauma, the theory helps us see these not as moral failings or weaknesses, but as innate responses coded into our nervous system meant to help us cope and survive.

Decades after its inception, the Polyvagal Theory continues to inspire a growing body of research, providing new insights in fields as diverse as mental health, trauma therapy, communication, and education. Through its emphasis on the profound interconnection between our physiology and psychology, the theory underscores the essence of our human experience—that we are, at our core, social beings wired for connection.

Understanding The Principles Of Polyvagal Theory

Delving into the principles of the Polyvagal Theory unveils a captivating narrative about our physiology and its influence on our emotions, behaviors, and social interactions. Three fundamental principles form the foundation of this theory, namely hierarchy, neuroception, and co-regulation.

The **hierarchical principle** refers to the ordered way in which our nervous system responds to our environment.

Imagine this hierarchy as a traffic light system. The green light corresponds to the Ventral Vagal Complex, the newest and most evolved part of our nervous system. It fosters social engagement and feelings of safety and calmness. The yellow light represents the Sympathetic Nervous System, an older system responsible for mobilization responses like fight-or-flight. Finally, the red light corresponds to the Dorsal Vagal Complex, the oldest part that governs immobilization responses such as freezing-or-fainting. This hierarchy elucidates how our body responds differently to varying degrees of perceived safety or threat.

The second principle, **neuroception**, is the term Porges coined to describe how our nervous system makes subconscious evaluations of safety, danger, or life-threat without requiring conscious awareness, which enables a much more speedy reaction. For instance, entering a warmly lit room filled with familiar faces can subconsciously trigger our neuroception of safety, activating our ventral vagal system and promoting feelings of calm and openness. In contrast, seeing a face that reminds us of an abuser, can immediately trigger our fight-or-flight response.

The final principle of the Polyvagal Theory is **co-regulation**, highlighting our biologically driven need for social interaction and connection. Co-regulation speaks to the way our physiological state can be influenced by the state of those around us. When we are in a safe and supportive social environment, our nervous system can mirror this safety, leading to feelings of calm, connectedness, and well-being. On the flip side, when someone else is on edge and nervous, we tend to replicate this state.

Grasping these principles of the Polyvagal Theory invites a profound shift in our understanding of ourselves. It provides a biological framework that explains why we react the way we do in different situations. The theory helps us realize that our physiological responses are not random or arbitrary; instead, they are guided by an intricate, adaptive, and deeply intelligent system aimed at ensuring our survival and often developed based on past experiences..

In essence, understanding the Polyvagal Theory is about gaining self-compassion and empathy towards our own and others' emotional states. It is about realizing that behind every emotional response, there is a physiological story unfolding, a story that connects us deeply to our human nature and to each other. Appreciating these stories allows the veil to drop and bring hidden responses into the consciousness.

The Autonomic Nervous System And The Polyvagal Theory

To truly appreciate the intricacies of the Polyvagal Theory, it is essential to explore its relationship with the autonomic nervous system (ANS). The ANS is a division of our peripheral nervous system responsible for regulating involuntary bodily functions such as heart rate, digestion, and respiratory rate. This behind-the-scenes maestro of our internal functions operates largely outside our conscious control. The ANS is divided into two primary subsystems, namely the sympathetic nervous system (SNS) and the parasympathetic nervous system (PNS), both of which the Polyvagal Theory helps illuminate.

The SNS, often associated with the fight-or-flight response, prepares the body for action in the face of perceived threats. It is like an internal alarm system that, when activated, results in increased heart rate, blood pressure, and alertness to quickly prepare us for potential danger. In the process, we do not have to activate the complex thinking center of our brain—the cerebral cortex.

On the other hand, the PNS, traditionally linked with rest-and-digest functions, promotes relaxation and restoration when the body perceives safety. It helps to slow heart rate, stimulate digestion, and conserve energy to maintain a state of calm and peace, and recuperate strength and wellbeing.

The Polyvagal Theory brings a refined understanding of the PNS by illustrating it as a two-tiered system, reflecting the dual branches of the vagus nerve as previously mentioned. The ventral vagal pathway, a myelinated branch, aligns with social engagement behaviors and feelings of safety. Conversely, the dorsal vagal pathway, an unmyelinated branch, is related to immobilization responses, like fainting, that are triggered when life-threatening situations are perceived.

All put together, this tripartite conception of the autonomic nervous system—ventral vagal (social engagement and calm), sympathetic (fight or flight), and dorsal vagal (immobilization)—provides a more nuanced understanding of our physiological and emotional responses. Rather than viewing the ANS as merely a system that vacillates between states of arousal and relaxation, the Polyvagal Theory unveils a more dynamic system finely attuned to our environment.

In this sense, the Polyvagal Theory is like a lens through which we can perceive the symphony of our autonomic functions. It enables us to realize that our nervous system is not just mechanically responding to internal and external stimuli but is constantly engaged in maintaining our wellbeing and promoting survival. Even if not perfectly balanced or adaptive, it is meant to protect us and help us cope. It is this understanding of our deeply interconnected physiology that invites us to approach our experiences with increased compassion, self-awareness, and resilience, helping us to achieve balance and adaptation.

Relevance Of Polyvagal Theory To Everyday Life

Embracing the Polyvagal Theory is not just about deepening our intellectual understanding of human physiology. Its real magic lies in its profound relevance and application to our everyday life. The theory offers a blueprint for understanding our emotional responses and provides practical tools for fostering resilience, enhancing communication, and nurturing healthier relationships.

One of the most transformative implications of the Polyvagal Theory is its ability to cultivate self-compassion and empathy. By recognizing that our emotional states are manifestations of our underlying physiological responses, we can better understand and accept our reactions to stressful or challenging situations. In an important sense, the Polyvagal Theory normalizes our emotional distress that affects our behavior. Instead of judging ourselves harshly for feeling anxious, stressed, or disconnected, we can extend kindness to ourselves, knowing that our bodies are just trying to keep us safe.

Moreover, the Polyvagal Theory can empower us to consciously influence our physiological state. Through practices such as deep breathing, mindfulness, and social connection, we can stimulate our ventral vagal system, the pathway linked to feelings of safety and social engagement. Over time, these practices can help us build physiological resilience and increase our capacity to navigate life's stressors with greater ease and equanimity.

In the context of relationships, the Polyvagal Theory underscores the importance of social connection and co-regulation. It reminds us that our nervous systems are inherently social and are continuously influenced by the physiological states of those around us. This understanding can inspire us to favor and foster safe, supportive, and nurturing relationships that can enhance our collective well-being.

Furthermore, the Polyvagal Theory can inform more effective communication. Recognizing the physiological underpinnings of our emotions can help us express our needs and feelings more accurately and empathetically without shame or embarrassment. This heightened emotional literacy can lead to deeper connections, increased understanding, and more satisfying interpersonal dynamics.

In essence, the Polyvagal Theory does not just pertain to the realms of neuroscience or psychology—it relates directly to the lived human experience. By offering a holistic, compassionate, and nuanced perspective of our physiology and emotional life, the theory equips us with a powerful framework for self-understanding, growth, and transformation.

2

— . —

UNDERSTANDING THE VAGUS NERVE AND ITS FUNCTIONS

I n the second chapter we go on a journey to understand the anatomical marvel that is the vagus nerve - a key player in our emotional and physiological well-being. The vagus nerve, also referred to as the "wandering nerve", is one of the longest cranial nerves in our body, boasting an extensive network of connections that play key roles in maintaining our wellbeing. The exploration of its functions will illuminate how intricately it is involved in regulating our heart rate, digestion, and even our emotional responses. As we unravel the importance of the vagus nerve within the framework of the Polyvagal Theory, we will delve into the concept of vagal tone and its significance in our lives.

Anatomy Of The Vagus Nerve

The name 'vagus' stems from the Latin word for 'wandering,' a fitting descriptor given the extensive reach of this nerve within our bodies The vagus nerve, also referred to as the tenth cranial nerve, begins its journey within the brainstem's medulla oblongata region. From there, it embarks on a long journey, descending down the neck and extending its branches throughout the body.

Left and right branches of the vagus nerve innervate various regions of the body. Their influence can be felt across organs such as heart, lungs, liver and digestive tract; making their reach both wide-reaching and profound. Remarkably, however, the vagus nerve is not only one way; both branches work simultaneously! It is a mixed nerve composed of both afferent (sensory) and efferent (motor) fibers.

Sensory fibers convey information from our bodies to the brain, such as organ function or stomach fullness. Meanwhile, motor fibers send messages back down from our minds directing organs to perform certain functions such as slowing heart rate or stimulating digestion. This bidirectional communication channel allows the vagus nerve to serve as a critical link between our brain and body.

Furthermore, the vagus nerve is unique in its composition. As highlighted in the Polyvagal Theory, the vagus is composed of two distinct pathways - the ventral and dorsal vagal pathways. The ventral vagal pathway, also known as the smart vagus, is myelinated, meaning it is coated with a fatty layer that enables faster signal transmission. In contrast, the dorsal vagal pathway is unmyelinated, leading to slower signal transmission. These dual branches play a significant role in our physiological and emotional responses, as we delve deeper into in the subsequent sections.

Functions Of The Vagus Nerve

The vagus nerve, in its wanderings, connects the brain with a host of vital organs in the body, facilitating crucial physiological functions. This vast network underlies the multitude of roles that the vagus nerve plays, making it instrumental in preserving our overall health and well-being.

The vagus nerve is best-known for its role in supporting the autonomic nervous system (ANS), particularly through the parasympathetic branch. The ANS, as we learned in Chapter 1, is responsible for the automatic bodily functions that happen without our conscious control - such as heartbeat, digestion, and respiration. The parasympathetic system, often referred to as the 'rest and digest' system, serves to conserve energy and maintain a state of calm in the body.

Here, the vagus nerve is at the forefront. Within the parasympathetic system, its primary role is regulating heart rate. In an ideal state of relaxation, when our body sends signals for it to slow its heartbeat down accordingly and promote a sense of calmness and relaxation. This function, called vagal tone, is crucial to our capacity to navigate stress and recovery.

Another critical area of influence of the vagus nerve is the digestive system. The vagal nerve plays a pivotal role in digestive processes, including food movement along the gut, production of digestive enzymes, regulation of hunger/satisfaction signals, and regulation of hunger/satisfaction signals. Therefore, disruptions in its function may result in various digestive issues including IBS or gastroparesis.

Further, the vagus nerve plays an integral part in regulating our breathing. It provides sensory feedback to the brain about lung inflation and controls the muscles involved in voice production and swallowing. Moreover, by stimulating the release of surfactants necessary for the lungs' functioning, it plays a role in neonatal respiratory adaptation at birth.

Perhaps, less known but equally important, the vagus nerve has immunomodulatory effects. Vagus nerve is an integral component of our body's anti-inflammatory response and known for activating what is referred to as the "cholinergic anti-inflammatory pathway", where vagus nerve signals the release of acetylcholine as neurotransmitter that helps dampen down inflammation response.

Finally, the vagus nerve contributes to our emotional responses and social engagement behaviors, playing a central role in the Polyvagal Theory. Emotional regulation is achieved via the connection between the vagus nerve and amygdala - two brain regions vitally involved with emotion processing - via vagal nerve reflex.

Indeed, the versatility and reach of the vagus nerve speak to the essential nature of its roles, ranging from those that are immediately palpable to those that subtly but continually maintain our well-being. The vagus nerve is our silent sentinel, continually monitoring and responding to changes in the internal environment and communicating these changes to our brain, facilitating appropriate responses. Understanding its functions allows us to fully appreciate its influence on our overall health and well-being.

In particular, the vagus nerve serves as an intermediary between conscious experiences and physical conditions. Its bidirectional communication function allows the brain to alter our bodily functions based on our psychological state and also provides feedback from our bodies to our minds. This interplay is of utmost significance in our experiences of emotion, stress, and social interactions.

As we delve further into the vagus nerve's role in the Polyvagal Theory in the following sections, this bidirectional mind-body connection becomes even more critical. It establishes the basis for understanding how we react emotionally and socially, providing insights into managing mental health conditions like anxiety, depression and PTSD. Thus, the vagus nerve, while being an essential physiological entity, is also a lynchpin in our emotional and social experiences.

As previously discussed, the vagus nerve is an indispensable part of our physical, psychological, emotional, and social wellbeing, serving an integral role in maintaining optimal physiological, emotional, and social well-being. Its functions range from the fundamentals of maintaining our physical health to the complexities of human emotional responses and social engagement behaviors. As we navigate the complex pathways of the vagus nerve, we gain not only knowledge of its basic functioning but also of how its underpinnings shape our emotional experiences and behaviors. The importance of the vagus nerve in our lives, as we shall see, extends far beyond its anatomical presence and biological functions.

The Vagus Nerve And Emotional Responses

The vagus nerve is more than an anatomical structure; it represents our bodies' delicate connection with mind, most notably when responding to emotional stimuli. The ability of the vagus nerve to influence and be influenced by our emotional states underpins its vital role in mental well-being and social engagement.

The connection between our vagus nerve and emotional responses lies within the bidirectional exchange between brain and body. Emotions, as we understand them, are not solely confined to the realms of our minds but are embodied experiences, with physical sensations often accompanying emotional states. The "butterflies" in the stomach before a big presentation or the rapid heartbeat during moments of fear are testimonies to this embodied nature of emotions. At this point, the vagus nerve plays an integral part. It transmits bodily sensations to our brains, shaping emotional experiences.

One key concept related to vagal tone refers to its activity level.. A higher vagal tone, associated with more frequent and robust vagus nerve activity, is linked to a greater capacity for emotional regulation. This is because a higher vagal tone enables faster and more effective engagement and disengagement of the parasympathetic nervous system, facilitating quicker recovery from stress and fostering emotional resilience.

On the flip side, a lower vagal tone, indicating less active vagus nerve functioning, is associated with difficulties in emotional regulation. Individuals with lower vagal tone may find it challenging to regulate their emotions effectively, resulting in an elevated stress response and potential negative emotional states such as anxiety and depression.

Vagus nerve's influence on emotional responses extends far beyond our internal emotional states. It extends to social engagement behaviors, including communication, empathy, and bonding. This is a significant part of the Polyvagal Theory, which proposes that the vagus nerve, particularly its ventral branch, is linked to the social engagement system. When active, this system facilitates feelings of safety, enabling social engagement behaviors and positive emotional states.

The vagus nerve also plays a role in the physiological responses associated with emotional experiences. This can range from changes in heart rate and respiration in response to stress, to the warm, relaxed feeling associated with social connection and feelings of safety. Therefore, the vagus nerve serves as a crucial link between our physiological state and emotional experiences.

Understanding how the vagus nerve influences our emotional experiences and responses can provide insights into physical manifestations of emotional states or disorders. For example, anxiety disorders often manifest physical symptoms such as rapid heartbeat, shortness of breath and gastrointestinal distress - symptoms which we know play an integral part in anxiety disorders' progression. We know now that the vagus nerve plays a crucial role in regulating bodily functions that play into anxiety disorder symptoms - disruptions can cause these physical manifestations. The relationship between physical and emotional is evidence of our interconnection between bodies and minds as we witness our bodies communicating their messages via vagus nerve.

The vagus nerve plays an integral part in both emotional and stress responses, helping the body return to a state of relaxation following stressful events through its parasympathetic nervous system. However, in individuals with a lower vagal tone, this 'rest and digest' response may be less efficient, leading to a prolonged stress response that can contribute to anxiety and other negative emotional states.

Vagus nerve not only plays an essential role in controlling negative emotional reactions, but it is also essential for experiencing positive ones - specifically those associated with social engagement and being connected. Studies have linked activating the vagus nerve to feelings of social connectedness and positive emotions. This is in line with the Polyvagal Theory's assertion that the vagus nerve is an integral part of the social engagement system.

As has become clear, the vagus nerve acts as a link between our physiological states and emotional experiences. It plays a significant role in emotional regulation, stress response and the experience of positive social connections and positive emotions - giving us greater appreciation of their holistic nature; emotions don't simply reside in our heads but throughout the body too!

Overall, the vagus nerve acts as an integral link between our bodies and minds, shaping emotional experiences and behaviors. This ability of the nerve to shape emotional responses highlights its essential role in mental health and well-being, providing the basis for therapeutic interventions designed to increase vagal tone for improved emotional regulation and social engagement. Understanding this connection can empower us to harness the power of the vagus nerve in managing our emotional health, fostering resilience, and enhancing our social relationships.

As stated above, the vagus nerve is not only an important physiological entity; its influence over emotional responses and body-mind connection makes it essential to emotional well-being. It provides a window into understanding our emotional lives more holistically, giving us the tools to manage our emotions effectively, foster resilience, and enhance our social relationships. Knowledge of this nature provides the basis for applying Polyvagal Theory in supporting mental health and well-being, which we will further examine in future chapters.

The Vagus Nerve And The Polyvagal Theory

According to Stephen Porges, the originator of the Polyvagal Theory, the vagus nerve is not a solitary unit but rather contains different fibers that are functionally differentiated. That means different aspects of the vagus nerve serve different roles, contributing to our bodies' complex responses in different circumstances. Understanding this complexity is essential to grasping the full implications of the Polyvagal Theory.

The Polyvagal Theory emphasizes the role of the vagus nerve in two primary physiological states - 'fight or flight' response and 'rest and digest' response. These states, controlled by the autonomic nervous system, allow us to react to environmental threats and then recover once the threat has passed. The vagus nerve, through its link with the parasympathetic nervous system, plays an integral part in supporting this recovery phase.

However, the vagus nerve is involved in both rest-and-digest responses as well as fight-flight reactions due to its dual myelinated-unmyelinated fiber composition. This facilitates its dual role. The myelinated vagal fibers are linked with the social engagement system, promoting calm states and social connection. In contrast, the unmyelinated vagal fibers, referred to as the 'dorsal vagal complex,' are associated with immobilization behaviors like fainting or 'playing dead,' which can be viewed as an extreme form of the 'fight or flight' response.

Porges suggests that these different vagal pathways can be activated under different circumstances, leading to different behavioral and physiological responses. For example, when we perceive a situation as safe, the myelinated vagal fibers can promote social engagement and feelings of calm. However, when we perceive extreme danger, the unmyelinated vagal fibers may become activated, leading to immobilization behaviors.

Implications of this understanding are far-reaching. It highlights that our bodies are equipped with nuanced and flexible systems for managing stress and danger. It also provides a physiological explanation for why we may respond differently to different forms of stressors, while emphasizing the vagus nerve's central role in mediating responses.

In essence, the vagus nerve is the physiological cornerstone of the Polyvagal Theory. Understanding its function, and the way in which it influences physiological and emotional responses, can empower us to harness its potential and improve our wellbeing.

The Importance Of Vagal Tone

In our exploration of the vagus nerve's functions and its role in the Polyvagal Theory, we have come across a critical concept – that of vagal tone. But what is vagal tone, and why is it significant within the context of Polyvagal Theory and our everyday lives?

Vagal tone refers to the activity of the vagus nerve. More specifically, vagal tone refers to the level of parasympathetic influence over the heart, which can be measured via heart rate variability (HRV). Simply stated, HRV measures how often time passes between heartbeats; higher HRV values (which indicates increased vagal tone) have been linked with improved health and well-being.

A high vagal tone, resulting in a greater HRV, reflects a robust and responsive autonomic nervous system. In practical terms, this means that a person with a higher vagal tone can adapt more effectively to stress, showing a swift and efficient 'fight or flight' response when needed and a rapid return to a 'rest and digest' state once the threat is no longer present. In contrast, a lower vagal tone suggests a less responsive autonomic nervous system, potentially leading to prolonged stress responses and difficulties in returning to a relaxed state.

Within the Polyvagal Theory, vagal tone is considered a key marker of the body's capacity to regulate physiological and emotional responses. Those with a higher vagal tone are typically better equipped to handle stress, engage socially, and maintain overall mental and physical health. This understanding provides a potential physiological explanation for variations in emotional resilience and social behavior among individuals.

The significance of vagal tone extends to various areas of life and health. Studies have associated higher vagal tone with numerous positive outcomes, including enhanced emotional regulation, greater social connectedness, decreased anxiety and depression levels and enhanced cognitive functioning. Conversely, low vagal tone has been linked with cardiovascular disease, stroke, mental health disorders and cognitive deficits.

In conclusion, the vagus nerve, a key player in the Polyvagal Theory, plays a multifaceted role in our lives. It helps regulate our bodies' functions, influences our emotional responses, and shapes our social interactions. Vagal tone has far-reaching implications for our health and well-being; understanding its functions and understanding its influence on human emotion are keys to making changes that align with our bodies' natural wisdom and lead to improved health, resilience, and social connections.

As we wrap up this chapter, it is crucial to reflect on how the intricate vagus nerve and its role within the Polyvagal Theory can influence our day-to-day lives. Understanding the fundamental functions of the vagus nerve, how it impacts our emotional responses, and how it interacts within the framework of the Polyvagal Theory, opens the door to optimizing our psychological and physiological well-being. Most importantly, recognizing the importance of vagal tone gives us the knowledge and tools to potentially influence our vagal tone, empowering us to manage stress effectively, engage socially, and maintain overall mental and physical health.

In the subsequent chapters, we will delve deeper into the practical applications of the Polyvagal Theory. The next chapter will focus on the connection between Polyvagal Theory and mental health. Thereafter, we will explore how this theory can be applied to improve communication and relationships, enhance performance, and integrate Polyvagal practices into daily life.

With this foundational understanding of the Polyvagal Theory and the vagus nerve, we are well-equipped to continue our exploration and begin applying these principles to our lives. The journey towards harnessing the power of the Polyvagal Theory to improve our relationships, performance, and over-all health is just beginning, and we have exciting discoveries awaiting us in the chapters to come.

3

— · —

THE CONNECTION BETWEEN THE POLYVAGAL THEORY AND MENTAL HEALTH

I n the third chapter of our journey into the Polyvagal Theory, we consider its touch points with mental health – an
essential and often misunderstood dimension of human life
and experience. Polyvagal Theory gives us the opportunity
to appreciate mental health as a result of both psychological
factors and physiological responses, of which are often instinctive and subconscious.

This knowledge gives us new insights into how our bodies, in
particular our nervous systems, influence our mental well-being. In this chapter, we explore the close relationship between
the Polyvagal Theory and various mental health conditions.
These include stress responses, anxiety disorders, depression,
and post-traumatic stress disorder (PTSD). With this information we help you understand your own mental health better.
In this and following chapters, we then provide you with the
tools to manage and enhance your well-being effectively.

Let's begin by examining how the Polyvagal Theory offers a
unique perspective on mental health.

The Polyvagal Perspective On Mental Health

In traditional views of mental health, such as the medical model that focuses on dysfunctions, psychological factors are often at the center. As a result, practitioners see distress in emotional experiences, thought processes, interpersonal relationships, and life events as the primary drivers of mental health conditions. But the Polyvagal Theory proposes a more integrated perspective, wherein mental health is seen not merely as a product of our minds but as a complex interaction between our mind and body, in other words, our psychological and physiological systems. From this perspective we can gain unique insights into our mental health, which open up new ways to improve our overall well-being.

Polyvagal Theory, which was developed by Dr. Stephen Porges in the 1990's, offers a compelling explanation of how our vagus nerve – an important part of the autonomic nervous system, plays a central role in our emotional and social experiences. The theory suggests that the vagus nerve is key to understanding our bodies' responses to stress and danger and how these responses can shape our mental health.

The autonomic nervous system comprises of the sympathetic and parasympathetic systems. Its role is to prepare our body to respond to threat or enable safety. In other words, the sympathetic system activates us for 'fight or flight', while the parasympathetic system encourages us to 'rest and digest,' or restoring our resources for when needed again.

Therefore, the vagus nerve plays a pivotal role in shifting us between these states, thereby maximizing our energy. However, if our bodies frequently enter into a state of high alert, or if they struggle to return to a relaxed state, we might experience mental health issues such as anxiety disorders, depression, and PTSD.

Polyvagal Theory also introduces the concept of 'neuroception,' which describes how our nervous system automatically scans our environment for cues of safety or danger. This unconscious surveillance can significantly impact our emotional state. If our neuroception detects threat, our body shifts into 'fight or flight' mode. This shift can be helpful in the short term but, when prolonged, frequent, or intense, can contribute to mental health issues by dysregulating the stress response system.

Furthermore, the Polyvagal Theory gives us a fresh perspective to how our social behavior impacts our mental health. According to Porges' theory, the vagus nerve enables or blocks us from connecting with others – a concept known as the 'social engagement system'. When our neuroception perceives safety, the social engagement system creates feelings of trust and calm, positively influencing our preference to connect and protecting our mental well-being.

To conclude, the Polyvagal perspective highlights the close links between our physiology and mental health. It emphasizes the importance of understanding our bodies' responses to stress and safety, the significance of our social engagement system, and the role of our autonomic nervous system in our mental well-being. As we further explore these connections in the following sections, we'll delve deeper into how this perspective can support our understanding and management of specific mental health conditions.

Polyvagal Theory And Stress Responses

Stress is an unavoidable part of human life. It is a natural, and often instinctive and automatic, reaction to prepare us to act, such as fight, flight, or freeze. These responses involve emotions, thoughts, and actions that happen very quickly to efficiently address any danger. When the stress is appropriate and relevant to our situation, it helps us stay alert, motivated, and ready to avoid danger. But it is unhelpful and harmful when it is sustained, or we overreact to something overestimated. Such chronic or acute stress is often the precipitate of mental health issues.

Here, the Polyvagal Theory explains how our body responds to stress and how these responses can be linked to our mental health. So, how does it work?

The sympathetic nervous system – a branch of our autonomic nervous system – activates when we perceive danger or stress. It prepares our bodies for a 'fight or flight' response with the objective to keep us safe and alive. The physiological changes like an elevated heart rate, blood pressure, and adrenaline levels enable us to act quickly to counter the threat.

Once the threat passes, the parasympathetic nervous system, primarily mediated by the vagus nerve, should ideally take over, calming the body and bringing it back to a state of 'rest and digest.'

However, problems can arise when our bodies are unable to shift back to this relaxed state due to constant stress or perceived threats, leading to what is known as chronic sympathetic activation. This chronic activation can result in mental health conditions like anxiety disorders and depression. The Polyvagal Theory suggests that if the vagus nerve's function is compromised, it might lead to difficulties in managing stress, leading to similar mental health outcomes.

This connection between stress responses and mental health underlines the importance of maintaining a healthy balance in our autonomic nervous system's activity. By nurturing our 'rest and digest' response and managing our 'fight or flight' response effectively, we can promote better mental health.

The Polyvagal perspective also highlights the importance of our bodies' ability to perceive safety, termed neuroception. When our neuroception continually perceives threat, even in the absence of real danger, it can contribute to chronic stress and anxiety. Understanding this concept can help us develop strategies to recalibrate our neuroception, encouraging it to perceive safety more often, thus alleviating chronic stress responses.

In the next few sections, we explore further how the Polyvagal Theory can be used to understand some of the more prevalent mental health conditions, including anxiety disorders, depression, and PTSD, which are closely linked to our bodies' stress responses. Therefore, understanding these links can provide us with valuable insights into managing these conditions more effectively.

Polyvagal Theory And Anxiety Disorders

Mood disorders, in particular anxiety and depression, are the most prevalent mental health conditions worldwide. They involve excessive and prolonged feelings of fear and anxiety that can significantly interfere with daily activities. The Polyvagal Theory offers a physiological perspective on these disorders, suggesting a link between the functioning of the vagus nerve and the symptoms of anxiety.

The Polyvagal Theory posits that most people presenting with anxiety disorders have an overactive sympathetic nervous system. As part of our autonomic nervous system that are responsible for our 'fight or flight' responses, this can result in a constant state of hyperarousal or vigilance that are not aligned with their real situation. As such, they suffer from symptoms like a racing heart, quick breathing, and feelings of restlessness and worry that are debilitating to their functioning.

Simultaneously, the theory proposes that these individuals might also have a compromised functioning of the vagus nerve, which plays a vital role in the parasympathetic nervous system's 'rest and digest' response. When functioning optimally, the vagus nerve should help calm the body down after a stressful event, reduce the heart rate, slow breathing, and create feelings of calm and relaxation. But if the vagus nerve's functioning is not healthy, individuals may struggle to 'switch off' their fight or flight response, contributing to chronic anxiety.

A key component of this link between the Polyvagal Theory and anxiety disorders is the concept of neuroception - our body's subconscious ability to detect safety or threat in our environment. In people with anxiety disorders, this neuroception might be skewed, leading them to perceive threats even in safe environments. This faulty neuroception can trigger an unwarranted 'fight or flight' response, manifesting as anxiety.

Understanding this Polyvagal perspective can lead to innovative approaches for managing anxiety disorders. For instance, therapies and exercises that promote vagal tone (the health of the vagus nerve) could be beneficial. These might include breathing exercises, mindfulness meditation, yoga, and even social interaction, as the theory suggests that feeling socially connected can also help activate our 'rest and digest' response.

Moreover, understanding this perspective can help individuals with anxiety disorders make sense of their experiences.

Knowing that their symptoms may be linked to their nervous system's responses can reduce self-blame and stigma. It also underscores the importance of nurturing a sense of safety – both physically and emotionally – as a strategy to manage anxiety.

In the next section, we explore how the Polyvagal Theory can be applied to understand another common mental health condition - depression.

Polyvagal Theory And Depression

Depression poses another significant global health concern characterized mainly by persistent negative feelings like hopelessness or sadness that trigger a lack of interest /pleasure during activities participated in . However, insight into possible treatment avenues yields through understanding depression's biological underpinnings by leveraging insights offered through The Polyvagal Theory.

An increasingly popular notion describes depression resulting from dysregulation issues fundamentally linked to an active parasympathetic nervous system - dominated by the vagus nerve. With this weakening comes an imbalanced response through reduced activation of 'rest-and-digest' mode leading to vulnerability towards fatalistic states influencing depressive symptoms.

Thus, the vagus nerve's contributions in mood regulation are highly crucial since it regulates production and release of mood-related neurotransmitters like serotonin and dopamine. Any disruption in this regulatory function could result in an imbalance incidence, commonly seen amongst individuals with depression. Additionally, such individuals often exhibit low vagal tone that limits their ability to disengage from stress or danger proactively.

Further findings attribute low vagal tone with poor emotional regulation alongside reduced resilience to stress - occurrences strongly linked to manifesting depressive symptoms similar to chronic "neural shutdown" responses.

Taking the Polyvagal Theory perspective towards addressing depression ought to emphasize improving patients' Vagal Tone through specific interventions like exercises aimed towards mindfulness, meditation, breathing techniques as well as improved social engagement activities. These interventions help enhance stress response regulation while promoting relaxation-response – leading towards alleviating and addressing depressive symptoms better.

Also having an enhanced appreciation for how depression intersects with Polyvagal Theory can benefit those living with this mental health condition as well as their caregivers in developing greater empathy while minimizing stigma. This viewpoint emphasizes that one's struggle with depression does not result from individual weaknesses or character defects. Rather it represents a natural response to life's deep-seated stresses which can be grasped, regulated and effectively treated. Subsequently we will explore how this theory correlates to PTSD in our next segment.

Polyvagal Theory And PTSD

Before concluding this chapter, it is important to examine how trauma impacts individuals both psychologically and physiologically.

Our attention turns specifically to Post Traumatic Stress Disorder (PTSD), a harmful disorder that frequently stems from experiencing traumatic events. It is characterized by recurrent, intrusive recollections of the event, avoidance of reminders, alterations in arousal and reactivity, and negative alterations in mood and cognitions. The Polyvagal Theory provides a unique framework for understanding how trauma can affect the body's physiology and result in the complex symptoms observed in PTSD.

In a traumatic situation, the body's safety system may fail to function properly. According to the Polyvagal Theory, the autonomic nervous system could get locked into a chronic state of 'fight or flight' (sympathetic dominance), or even into the more primitive 'freeze' response (dorsal vagal dominance).

This chronic dysregulation can manifest in numerous ways, such as hypervigilance, a common symptom where the person is excessively aware of signs of danger. Other symptoms include chronic anxiety, insomnia, and emotional dysregulation.

Further, trauma can also disrupt the body's ability to detect safety, impairing social engagement behaviors, and leading to feelings of disconnection or isolation - common in individuals with PTSD. Here, the Polyvagal Theory underscores the significance of social bonds and perceived safety in our environment for maintaining mental well-being.

The Polyvagal Theory also points towards novel therapeutic avenues for PTSD. Interventions aimed at restoring autonomic regulation, such as trauma-sensitive yoga or certain types of body-based psychotherapy, have shown promise. These practices can help rebalance the autonomic nervous system, promote feelings of safety, and aid recovery.

In sum, the Polyvagal Theory offers not just a powerful lens to understand mental health conditions like anxiety, depression, and PTSD but also informs novel and effective strategies for their treatment. By considering the biophysiological roots of these disorders, the theory facilitates a more compassionate and holistic approach to mental health.

FREE GOODWILL

D ear inquisitive mind,

I want to take a moment to recognize the enormous worth of your viewpoint and thoughts as you explore deeper into this book. For individuals looking for comfort, understanding, and a way to recover, your views and experiences can serve as a ray of hope.

I kindly ask you to take advantage of the chance to share your experience by giving this book an honest review.

Your review has the potential to empower people who may be dealing with trauma, anxiety, or a chronic condition. It is not just a simple opportunity for you to express your opinions. Your comments can offer consolation, direction, and a fresh sense of possibilities.

Let's work together to create a welcoming environment where compassion and empathy can flourish. Sharing your thoughts opens up a space for people to find comfort and affirmation in their experiences.

I want to thank you from the bottom of my heart for being willing to add to our understanding of the Polyvagal Theory. Your review will act as a lighthouse in helping others navigate the complex web of trauma, anxiety, chronic illness, and mental stress. Your words have power and the power to inspire change and give people hope.

I wish you a transforming journey of self-discovery and healing as you investigate the amazing discoveries of the Polyvagal Theory.

Sincere regards.

4

--- · ---

APPLYING POLYVAGAL THEORY TO IMPROVE COMMUNICATION AND RELATIONSHIPS

I n the fourth chapter, we shift our focus to the practical application of the Polyvagal Theory in our day-to-day interactions and relationships. Without applying theory in practice, we lose the value of our new insights. Understanding our physiological responses through the lens of the Polyvagal Theory can profoundly enhance our communication skills, our ability to empathize with others, and our capacity for resolving conflicts. It also offers insights that can help us build secure and fulfilling relationships. The following sections delve into each of these aspects, offering not only an in-depth understanding but also practical strategies and exercises to empower you in enriching your social connections and interactions.

The Polyvagal Theory And Emotion Regulation

The Polyvagal Theory opens up a new realm of understanding when it comes to emotional regulation, offering us a physiological perspective on why we feel what we feel and how we can better manage our emotional states. Emotional regulation is the process by which individuals influence which emotions they have, when they have them, and how they experience and express these emotions. It is a critical component of our mental well-being and plays a significant role in our interactions and relationships.

According to the Polyvagal Theory, our emotional responses are closely tied to the functioning of our autonomic nervous system and particularly the vagus nerve. As explained in earlier chapters, our nervous system operates on a hierarchy of responses – social engagement (ventral vagal complex), 'fight or flight' (sympathetic nervous system), and 'freeze or shut down' (dorsal vagal complex) responses. These responses are automatic and are influenced by our inclined state of mind and perception of safety or threat in our environment.

In the context of emotional regulation, this understanding is empowering. It tells us that our emotions are not something abstract, arbitrary, or entirely under the sway of conscious control. Instead, they are part of an adaptive response system designed to help us navigate our environment effectively, primarily to thrive, cope, or survive. For instance, feelings of anxiety may be linked to our body's 'fight or flight' response, while feelings of disconnection or numbness may be associated with the freeze response. When we perceive our environment as safe, we are more likely to feel calm, connected, and open to social engagement.

So, how can we use this understanding to enhance our emotional regulation? A key strategy is to cultivate a sense of safety, both internally and in our environment. Internal safety can be developed through practices like mindful breathing, meditation, or yoga, which have been found to stimulate the vagus nerve and promote a state of 'rest and digest'. On the other hand, environmental safety can be nurtured by building supportive relationships, creating a soothing, secure, and comfortable physical environment, and developing routines that provide predictability and stability.

Moreover, by understanding our emotional reactions as part of our body's adaptive response system, we can approach our feelings with greater compassion and curiosity, rather than judgment, fear, or shame. This shift in perspective can make it easier for us to explore our emotions, understand their roots, and navigate them more effectively.

In summary, the Polyvagal Theory provides us with a map to understand our emotional landscape and offers us practical strategies to enhance our emotional regulation. In the following sections, we look deeper into how these insights can be applied to improve communication and relationships.

The Role Of Polyvagal Theory In Building Empathy

Empathy, the capacity to understand and share the feelings of others, is a cornerstone of successful interpersonal relationships. It enables us to connect deeply with others, build rapport, and foster mutual understanding. The Polyvagal Theory offers a fascinating physiological perspective on empathy and gives us tools to enhance our empathetic responses.

According to Polyvagal Theory, our capacity for empathy is closely tied to the functioning of our ventral vagal complex, which supports social engagement and feelings of connection. When we feel safe and our ventral vagal system is active, we are more open to social engagement and more capable of empathy and trust. Conversely, when we perceive threat and our 'fight or flight' or freeze responses are activated, our capacity for empathy is diminished as our priority becomes safety and survival.

This physiological understanding helps explain why we might struggle with empathy in certain situations. For instance, during times of high stress, our body is more likely to be in a 'fight or flight' state, making it harder for us to connect empathetically with others. Similarly, if we have experienced trauma or prolonged periods of stress, our body might be prone to a freeze response, which can also inhibit our ability to empathize.

Understanding this can help us be more compassionate with ourselves and others when empathy feels challenging. It can also guide us towards strategies to enhance our capacity for empathy. Just as with emotional regulation, one of the key strategies here is to cultivate a sense of safety. By engaging our ventral vagal system through practices like deep, slow breathing, mindfulness, or soothing self-talk, we can shift our body towards a state that is more conducive to empathy.

Additionally, Polyvagal Theory suggests that our capacity for empathy can be enhanced by practicing attunement to the physiological states of others. This is based on the concept of 'neuroception,' a term coined by Dr. Stephen Porges to describe how our nervous system intuitively perceives the physiological states of others and responds accordingly. By becoming more attuned to the subtle cues indicating others' emotional states – such as tone of voice, facial expression, and body language – we can better understand their feelings and respond empathetically.

Finally, it is worth noting that empathy is not just about understanding others' feelings; it also involves communicating that understanding. The Polyvagal Theory highlights the importance of non-verbal communication in this regard, such as maintaining eye contact, mirroring body language, and using a warm, gentle tone of voice. Such cues can help signal safety to others' nervous systems, making it easier for them to open up and feel understood. In this way we achieve co-regulation – reciprocally sending and receiving cues of safety – by recognizing and resonating with the vagal tone of another person.

In conclusion, the Polyvagal Theory provides a unique physiological perspective on empathy, linking it closely with our perception of safety and the functioning of our autonomic nervous system. By using these insights, we can cultivate our empathetic responses, enhancing our relationships and interpersonal interactions.

Polyvagal Theory In Conflict Resolution

Conflict is an inevitable part of human relationships, but how we handle these conflicts defines the quality of our interactions and relationships. The Polyvagal Theory offers invaluable insights into conflict resolution, highlighting the vital role of our nervous system's responses in the way we perceive and manage disagreements.

When we are engaged in conflict, our body's response can often mimic that of a perceived threat. Our sympathetic nervous system, which controls the 'fight-or-flight' response, may be triggered, leading to heightened tension and a potential escalation of the conflict. Here, Polyvagal Theory provides an enlightening perspective. By being aware of and understanding our physiological responses during conflicts, we can develop strategies to manage situations more effectively.

In essence, to resolve conflict constructively, we need to shift from a state of 'fight-or-flight' (or freeze, for that matter) to a state of social engagement, as governed by the ventral vagal system, which is not always the intuitive choice. When our ventral vagal system is active, we are in a state of safety and connectedness, and we are better able to communicate, listen, and collaborate—skills that are crucial for effective conflict resolution.

So, how can we make this shift? One strategy involves switching on an internal sense of safety. When we feel threatened during a conflict, our immediate reaction might be to defend our stance aggressively (fight) or withdraw from the conversation (flight or freeze). However, by using self-regulation techniques such as deep, slow breathing, a mindful state of mind, or self-soothing talk, we can help ourselves feel safer and more grounded. This can create the space we need to respond to the conflict in a more thoughtful, constructive manner by engaging the prefrontal cortex, the thinking center of our brain instead of being purely reactive.

In addition, we can use our understanding of the Polyvagal Theory to help create a safer environment for conflict resolution. This involves using non-verbal cues such as maintaining eye contact, using a calm voice, and adopting a non-threatening body language, which can help signal safety to the other person's nervous system. It is also important to listen attentively and validate the other person's feelings, as this can help them feel heard and understood, further promoting a sense of safety.

Moreover, the concept of 'co-regulation' in Polyvagal Theory can be very useful in conflict resolution. As previously mentioned, co-regulation refers to the process of our nervous systems mutually influencing each other in social interactions. By consciously trying to maintain a calm and composed state during a conflict, we can potentially help 'co-regulate' the other person's nervous system, making it easier for them to also shift from a 'fight-or-flight' response to a state of social engagement.

In summary, the Polyvagal Theory provides a powerful framework for understanding and managing conflicts more effectively. By recognizing and responding to our physiological reactions, and by fostering a sense of safety and connection, we can approach conflicts in a way that promotes constructive resolution and enhances our relationships.

Cultivating Secure Attachments With Polyvagal Theory

Our relationships and connections form the basis of our emotional health, influencing our sense of self, well-being, and even our capacity to thrive in life. Attachment theory, an important area of psychological research, posits that our early experiences of bonding with our caregivers create a blueprint for future relationships. Within this context, the Polyvagal Theory introduces a fresh and physiologically grounded perspective on how to cultivate secure attachments in our relationships.

Secure attachment is characterized by a feeling of safety, comfort, and trust in relationships, which translates into openness, authentic connection, and balanced independence. As per the Polyvagal Theory, our capacity to form such secure attachments is closely tied to the functioning of the ventral vagal system. When this system is activated, it fosters a state of social engagement, where we are attuned to social cues, can express empathy, and are better able to communicate and connect with others.

Cultivating secure attachments, therefore, involves stimulating the ventral vagal system, thereby encouraging a shift towards the social engagement state. One strategy to achieve this is through co-regulation, a process in which two people's nervous systems mutually influence each other during social interaction. For example, using a calm and soothing voice, maintaining eye contact, or using touch (if appropriate), can help promote feelings of safety and connection in the other person, effectively aiding in activating their ventral vagal system too.

Another approach is to nurture our internal sense of safety, which is also fundamental to secure attachment. This can be achieved once more by practicing self-regulation techniques like deep, mindful breathing, grounding exercises, or self-soothing talk. These practices help to manage our stress responses, allowing us to stay calm and composed during interactions, thereby fostering more secure and healthy connections.

Interestingly, the Polyvagal Theory also suggests that our capacity to form secure attachments can be enhanced by improving our vagal tone – the activity level of the vagus nerve. Higher vagal tone is associated with better emotional regulation, increased resilience to stress, and more positive social behavior – all factors that contribute to secure attachment. Techniques for improving vagal tone range from practices like yoga, mindful practices, and regular physical activity, to specific biofeedback techniques where the effects of relaxing and purposeful activities are monitored and serve as reinforcement to secure states.

In sum, the Polyvagal Theory offers unique insights and practical strategies for cultivating secure attachments in our relationships. By understanding and working with our physiological responses, we can foster a sense of safety, connection, and social engagement, which are foundational for secure attachment and fulfilling relationships.

Practical Strategies For Applying Polyvagal Principles In Communication

As we continue to explore different realms of the Polyvagal Theory, it becomes evident that this biological framework is not merely of theoretical or academic interest. Instead, it holds practical relevance and can be applied in our daily lives, especially in the sphere of interpersonal communication. By utilizing Polyvagal principles, we can foster more effective, empathetic, and fulfilling interactions. This section outlines some practical strategies for applying the Polyvagal Theory in everyday communication.

- **Cultivating Mindful Awareness** - As we have discovered, our bodily states play a pivotal role in our social interactions. By cultivating mindful awareness, we can tune into our body's cues and become more attuned to shifts in our autonomic state. Recognizing these shifts enables us to respond effectively to our emotional needs, which can significantly enhance the quality of our communication. This means to be purposefully mindful and attentive to everything we do and experience.

- **Developing Emotional Regulation Techniques** - Emotional regulation plays a crucial role in effective communication. Techniques that stimulate the ventral vagal system, such as deep breathing, meditation, or even humming, can help us maintain a state of calm and composure during interactions, thereby promoting healthier communication. Practice recognizing, labeling, and accepting different emotions.

- **Fostering Co-Regulation** - Co-regulation is a key concept in Polyvagal Theory. It refers to the process of our nervous systems interacting and influencing each other during social engagement. By being mindful of our body language, tone of voice, and other non-verbal cues, we can foster co-regulation and enhance our connections with others, while acknowledging and tuning into their vagal tone.

- **Building Social Engagement Skills** - Polyvagal Theory emphasizes the importance of the social engagement system in healthy relationships and effective communication. Building skills such as active listening, expressing empathy, and demonstrating understanding can help activate the social engagement system, fostering more satisfying and meaningful interactions.

- **Enhancing Vagal Tone** - As discussed in the previous chapters, enhancing vagal tone can help improve emotional regulation, resilience, and social engagement - all of which are essential for effective communication. Regular exercise, yoga, meditation, laughter, and other joint experiences are some of the practices that can contribute to a higher vagal tone.

By integrating these strategies into our daily interactions, we can harness the power of the Polyvagal Theory to improve our communication skills and enhance our relationships. As we close this chapter, it is essential to remember that these practices are not a quick fix or a one-size-fits-all solution. They require patience, persistence, and compassion towards ourselves and others. But the reward—a richer, more meaningful connection with ourselves and those around us—is undoubtedly worth the effort.

5

LEVERAGING POLYVAGAL THEORY FOR PERFORMANCE ENHANCEMENT

I n the arena of human performance - whether at work, in sports, in academia, or even in the routine tasks of daily life - a nuanced understanding of our physiological responses can be a game changer. As we strive to excel in our respective domains, managing stress, maintaining focus, building resilience, and regulating energy become critical areas of interest. This is where the Polyvagal Theory, with its intricate understanding of the human nervous system and its responses, comes into play. In this chapter, we will delve deeper into how the Polyvagal Theory can be leveraged for enhancing our performance in various spheres of life. Let's begin our exploration by looking at how the Polyvagal Theory provides valuable insights into effective stress management.

Let's move onto the first subject area, which is how to manage stress to improve performance.

The Polyvagal Theory And Stress Management

One of the fundamental benefits of understanding the Polyvagal Theory is its utility in stress management. As we have alluded to before, stress, in its simplest definition, is our body's response to any demand placed upon it, whether physical, mental, or emotional. However, not all stress is harmful. It is our body's way of preparing us to face a challenge, to adapt, to survive. 'Eustress,' is the positive kind of stress that enhances our performance and keeps us alert and focused. On the converse, there is 'distress,' the negative type of stress, which, when persistent, increases the risk to develop various mental and physical health issues.

In the context of the Polyvagal Theory, stress triggers an immediate physiological response in our body by signals between brain and body through the vagus nerve. If we perceive a threat, whether real or imagined, our autonomic nervous system (ANS), more specifically our sympathetic nervous system, is activated. This response, often referred to as the 'fight or flight' mode, readies us to either confront the situation or escape from it. On the other hand, when the perceived threat is too overwhelming, our body may trigger the 'freeze' or 'shutdown' response, a survival mechanism primarily governed by the dorsal vagal complex of the parasympathetic nervous system.

Understanding these stress responses can enable effective stress management. By being aware of our body's physiological responses to stress, we can learn to identify the triggers that shift us into a sympathetic state or even a dorsal vagal state. This awareness can signal the need for an intervention that guides us to a more balanced state, a process known as 'self-regulation.' The ultimate goal of stress management, in the context of the Polyvagal Theory, is to stay in, or return to, the ventral vagal state as much as possible, which is the state of safety and social engagement.

Self-regulation can be enacted in various forms that range from deep breathing exercises that stimulate the vagus nerve to activities that promote social connection and feelings of safety. The key is to consciously work towards activating our parasympathetic nervous system, which promotes the 'rest and digest' or 'tend and befriend' responses. This helps counteract the effects of distress and brings our body back to a state of calm and balance.

It is worth noting that our ability to self-regulate does not mean completely avoiding the activation of the sympathetic nervous system or the dorsal vagal complex. Instead, it is about fostering a dynamic balance in our ANS, where we can smoothly transition between different states based on the demands of the environment. In simpler terms, this means that we need to take time to observe and think to objectively gauge any threat to determine the best response.

In summary, the Polyvagal Theory offers a physiological framework for understanding our stress responses. It provides us with the tools to become more aware of our body's signals and recognize triggers, so that we can effectively manage our reactions to stress, and ultimately enhance our performance by maintaining a balanced state that offers us more energy when needed and a clearer mind.

Polyvagal Theory And Focus

The human ability to maintain focus and attention is not just a cognitive process; it is also closely linked to our physiological state, something that is addressed in Polyvagal Theory. Our ability to pay attention, sustain focus, and manage distractions significantly impact our performance, whether in an academic, professional, or personal setting. Consequently, understanding the role of the Polyvagal Theory in these aspects provides valuable insights into how we can enhance our concentration and thereby improve our performance.

As such, the Polyvagal Theory helps us understand that our nervous system is continually responding to signals from the environment, forever shifting us between different states of the autonomic nervous system. When we are in a safe and socially connected state, known as the ventral vagal state, we are more capable of sustained attention and focus. In contrast, when our nervous system shifts us into a state of fight or flight or freeze, it can become much more challenging to maintain focus.

The reason for this difference lies in the evolutionary purpose of these different states. When our nervous system perceives a threat, it prioritizes survival over cognitive processes like thinking, focus, and attention. Our bodies prepare to either fight the threat or flee from it. These are processes that require rapid and instinctive action rather than contemplative thought and conscious decision-making. Even in the freeze or shut down state, our cognitive resources are focused more on automatic internal regulation rather than thoughtful external focus.

But when we are in a safe and socially connected state, our nervous system enables us to engage in more complex cognitive processes. Our bodies are not in a heightened state of alert for danger, freeing up our cognitive resources to concentrate on the task at hand. This means that when we're in the ventral vagal state, the thinking center of our brain, the prefrontal cortex are engaged, As a result, we are generally better equipped to manage distractions, sustain attention, and stay focused on a single task.

Understanding this connection between our physiological state and our ability to focus provides us with valuable tools to manage our attention. By learning to recognize which state we are in at any moment, we can begin to influence our physiological state and thereby our cognitive processes. For instance, if we find it challenging to concentrate, it might be an indication that we are in a state of 'fight or flight' or freeze. In such a case, using strategies to shift into the ventral vagal state could help enhance our focus. For example, when becoming aware of distress, taking a moment to step away from the perceived threat may restore objective focus and calm.

Furthermore, the regular practice of certain activities, such as deep, slow breathing, yoga, or mindfulness, which are known to promote a shift towards the ventral vagal state, can also help enhance our ability to focus. By incorporating such practices into our routine, we can potentially improve our attention regulation and thereby our overall performance.

Overall, the Polyvagal Theory offers a unique perspective on focus and attention, emphasizing that our cognitive processes are deeply interconnected with our physiological state and tend to disconnect when under acute stress. By understanding and harnessing this connection, we can create an environment that is conducive to sustained attention and high performance.

Resilience And Polyvagal Theory

Resilience is a vital characteristic, as it defines our ability to recover from setbacks, adapt to change, and keep going in the face of adversity. It is particularly important in today's fast-paced and highly stressful world, where we are often faced with challenges and obstacles. So, how does the Polyvagal Theory contribute to our understanding of resilience, and how can we use its principles to enhance our own resilience?

The Polyvagal Theory, with its emphasis on the body's automatic responses to environmental stressors, indeed provides a unique and insightful perspective on resilience that we can use to make our performance more robust. According to this theory, resilience is not just a product of our mindset or conscious efforts but is deeply rooted in our physiological responses to stress and danger. In simpler terms, the ability to thoughtfully react to one's environment reinforces resilience.

The ventral vagal complex (VVC), which is associated with the social engagement system, plays a crucial role in resilience. When we feel safe, the VVC is active, promoting social engagement, positive emotions, and healthy physiological states. This allows us to respond flexibly to life's challenges, bounce back from setbacks, and maintain a positive outlook. However, under severe stress or threat, the VVC can become deactivated, leading to a state of 'fight or flight' (associated with the sympathetic nervous system) or 'freeze' (associated with the dorsal vagal complex).

In this way, the Polyvagal Theory links resilience to the state of our autonomic nervous system. Therefore, enhancing our resilience involves improving our physiological capacity to maintain or return to the 'safe' state associated with the VVC, even under stress. This is where the concept of vagal tone, which we discussed in previous chapters, comes into play. A higher vagal tone is associated with better emotion regulation, social engagement, and stress management - all key elements of resilience.

The Polyvagal Theory also provides an explanation for why social support is so vital for resilience. According to the theory, social engagement, characterized by facial expressiveness, vocal communication, and feelings of safety in relationships, stimulates the VVC and helps maintain a physiological state conducive to resilience through safety and purpose. This is one of the reasons why individuals with a strong social network often demonstrate higher resilience in the face of adversity.

But how can we apply this knowledge to enhance our own resilience? One approach is to work on enhancing our vagal tone, which can be achieved through practices like mindful breathing, yoga, and meditation. Additionally, fostering meaningful social connections and working on our communication skills, as suggested in the previous chapter, can also help stimulate the VVC and promote resilience. Lastly, recognizing when we are in a 'fight or flight' or 'freeze' state and using self-regulation strategies to return to a 'safe' state can be a powerful tool for building resilience.

In summary, the Polyvagal Theory provides a physiological perspective on resilience, emphasizing the role of the autonomic nervous system and particularly the VVC in our ability to bounce back from adversity. By understanding these principles, we can take concrete steps to enhance our own resilience, helping us to navigate life's challenges more effectively.

The Role Of Polyvagal Theory In Energy Regulation

The concept of energy regulation might seem fuzzy, but it is a critical component of performance. Energy, in this context, refers to our physical, mental, and emotional resources that we utilize throughout the day to meet the demands of our lives. In a state of optimal energy regulation, we experience a sense of vitality, alertness, and readiness to engage with our environment. Conversely, when energy regulation is disrupted, we might feel fatigued, demotivated, frustrated, or overwhelmed. This is another area where the Polyvagal Theory provides useful insights.

At its core, the theory posits that our autonomic nervous system, and more specifically our vagus nerve, plays a crucial role in our body's energy regulation. Remember that the vagus nerve is part of our body's 'rest-and-digest system,' which helps to conserve energy, promote healing, and maintain homeostasis. When we're in a state of safety or social engagement, the myelinated vagus nerve (the component of the ventral vagal complex) helps to keep our energy expenditure in check, enabling us to rest, rejuvenate, and restore our energy reserves.

However, when we perceive danger or threat, our autonomic nervous system shifts towards a 'fight-or-flight' response, overseen by the sympathetic nervous system. This response is energy-intensive, as it requires rapid mobilization of resources, such as blood supply and adrenaline, to cope with the perceived threat. Especially when sustained, activation of the 'fight-or-flight' response can lead to energy depletion, chronic stress, and ultimately burnout, significantly impairing our performance.

Therefore, understanding the Polyvagal Theory can help us recognize when our energy regulation is off-balance and guide us in restoring equilibrium. For instance, signs of being stuck in the 'fight-or-flight' mode might include chronic tension, difficulty relaxing, and persistent feelings of restlessness or agitation. By applying the same Polyvagal-informed strategies such as deep breathing, social connection, and mindful self-regulation, we can stimulate the myelinated vagus nerve to bring our system back into a state of rest and digest, facilitating optimal energy regeneration and regulation.

Moreover, the Polyvagal Theory can help us become more attuned to our body's subtle signals of energy depletion, enabling us to take proactive steps to rest and recharge before hitting the point of exhaustion. In short, we are more attentive to recognize cues of a lack of energy and understand where it comes from. It highlights the importance of maintaining a balance between activity and rest, and between engagement and disengagement, in managing our energy levels effectively.

In essence, the Polyvagal Theory offers a powerful framework for understanding and managing our energy regulation, contributing to enhanced performance across various domains of life. By tuning into our body's cues and aligning with our innate physiological rhythms, we can optimize our energy regulation, fostering greater vitality, resilience, and well-being.

Practical Strategies For Performance Enhancement Through Polyvagal Principles

As mentioned before, practice must follow theory. It is only through action based on understanding that we reap the benefits. Translating the insights of the Polyvagal Theory into concrete actions can lead to performance enhancement in multiple areas of life. Let's explore some practical strategies grounded in the principles of the Polyvagal Theory to effectively manage stress, improve focus, build resilience, and regulate energy, thereby optimizing performance.

- **Mindful Breathing** - Deep, slow, and rhythmic breathing is one of the simplest and most effective strategies to activate the ventral vagal complex, and promoting a sense of calm, focus, and equilibrium. This kind of mindful breathing can be particularly beneficial before engaging in tasks that require high concentration or dealing with challenging situations.

- **Grounding Techniques** - Grounding is a set of techniques aimed at helping you reconnect with the present moment, often through focusing on physical sensations. This can help counteract the disorienting effects of stress and anxiety, enhancing focus and presence. Examples include mindfulness meditation, progressive muscle relaxation, and nature walks while focusing on your sensory experiences.

- **Social Connection** - As the Polyvagal Theory emphasizes, the ventral vagal complex is heavily involved in social engagement. Regular, meaningful social interactions stimulate this system, promoting feelings of safety, reducing stress, and enhancing overall well-being. Make time for social activities that you enjoy and that foster positive connections.

- **Regular Physical Activity** - Moderate exercise is a potent stimulator of the ventral vagal complex, helping to manage stress and maintain energy levels. Regular physical activity can improve mood, increase focus, and boost overall performance.

- **Balanced Nutrition** - Our diet can significantly influence the functioning of the nervous system. Consuming a balanced diet rich in fruits, vegetables, lean proteins, and healthy fats can support optimal neurological function and energy regulation.

- **Adequate Rest and Recovery** - As the Polyvagal Theory highlights, rest is a crucial part of maintaining balance in our autonomic nervous system and conserving energy. Ensure you are getting sufficient sleep and taking regular breaks during periods of work or study to allow your system to rejuvenate.

Applying these Polyvagal-informed strategies requires regular practice and self-compassion. While not expecting changes to happen overnight, remember that consistency will lead to noticeable improvements in stress management, focus, resilience, and energy regulation, ultimately enhancing performance.

To conclude, the Polyvagal Theory offers a robust framework to understand and enhance human performance. By leveraging its principles, we can better understand and recognize our physiological responses to different situations, learn to manage our energy levels more effectively, and cultivate practices that lead to better stress management, improved focus, and greater resilience. In short, understanding and applying the principles of the Polyvagal Theory can significantly improve our ability to perform and succeed in different aspects of life.

6

INTEGRATING POLYVAGAL PRACTICES INTO DAILY LIFE

As previously indicated, the power of Polyvagal Theory lies not only in its insights into our nervous system's inner workings but more so in its practical applications for everyday life. This chapter aims to empower you with knowledge and techniques to effectively utilize the principles of the Polyvagal Theory in your routine. We explore the essence of Polyvagal practices, delve into exercises that enhance vagal tone, introduce mindfulness strategies rooted in Polyvagal Theory, discuss applications for sleep and relaxation, and finally, guide you on integrating these practices seamlessly into your daily life. By applying the power of the Polyvagal Theory, you can actively contribute to your physical health, emotional stability, and overall well-being.

Understanding Polyvagal Practices

Polyvagal practices refer to the application of Polyvagal Theory principles in tangible, actionable ways that help manage stress, improve emotional regulation, and promote a sense of safety and social connection. The theory's core emphasis is on understanding the body's physiological responses, enabling you to consciously influence them to enhance well-being. These practices engage our biology, which leverage our body's built-in mechanisms for self-soothing and regulation.

By engaging our social engagement system - the branch of our nervous system associated with feelings of safety, relaxation, and social interaction - Polyvagal practices aim to tip the balance away from defensive states (fight, flight, freeze) towards a state of calm and connection. These activities can take many forms, including specific breathing techniques, mindfulness exercises, physical activities, and ways of enhancing social interaction.

One fundamental idea underpinning these practices is the notion of 'neuroception' – our nervous system's automatic, subconscious detection of safety or danger. By understanding our neuroception, we can influence it, thereby better managing our body's responses to the world around us. The goal is not to eliminate stress or avoid negative experiences - as these are inevitable parts of life - but to enhance our capacity to navigate them effectively and recover quickly and thoroughly in order to enhance performance and enhance happiness.

Practices For Enhancing Vagal Tone

New possibilities of well-being open up when you start to understand the significance of the vagus nerve and its tone in your life. The term 'vagal tone' points to the health and function of your vagus nerve. It is about how effectively this important nerve can perform its duties, which ultimately impact your physical health, your ability to regulate emotions, and your resilience to stress. As your vagus nerve health improves, so too will its vagal tone and overall well-being. So, the question you are probably asking is – how can one enhance their vagal tone? The good news is that we are about to share several strategies that can assist you on this journey.

Deep Breathing

One of the easiest and most effective ways to stimulate and increase vagal tone is through deep, mindful breathing. Your respiratory system and vagus nerve share a special connection, so this approach may work especially well in stimulating this nerve.

As you take slow, deep breaths, it acts like you are sending a relaxing signal directly to the vagus nerve. The nerve responds, in turn, by helping your body switch to a state of relaxation.

You can try this practice of mindful, diaphragmatic breathing daily.

Place yourself in a peaceful environment and focus on your breathing. Inhale slowly through your nose, then exhale gently out through your mouth. Do not focus on how many breaths you take every minute; rather try breathing in deeply and mindfully as much as possible.

Physical Exercise

Physical exercise is another effective way of enhancing your vagal tone. Regular moderate-intensity physical activity such as walking, swimming or cycling can have an incredible effect on vagal tone. It does so by altering heart rate and blood pressure - two vital variables controlled by the vagus nerve. Interestingly, it is not about exercising intensively but more about maintaining a regular, moderate level of physical activity that is typically more beneficial for your vagal tone.

Social Interaction

In third place, let us not forget the powerful role of social interaction as a way of enhancing our vagal tone. The vagus nerve is a crucial part of our social engagement system, and positive, supportive interactions can stimulate it. Engaging in social activities that bring joy, spending quality time with loved ones, building and maintaining positive social connections - all of these can contribute to a higher vagal tone.

Mindfulness And Meditation

Yoga, Tai Chi, and meditation are all forms of mind-body practices that can work wonders for your vagal tone. These practices often combine controlled breathing, physical postures, and mental focus - a trifecta that promotes relaxation, relieves stress, and activates the vagus nerve. Implementing any of these practices into your routine can greatly enhance vagal tone, leading to improved emotional balance, stress resilience and overall well-being.

In our journey through life, understanding and working with our body's natural systems can be the key to unlocking a better version of ourselves. These practices for enhancing vagal tone offer just such an opportunity. As you incorporate these into your daily routine, you would be embracing a path towards personal growth and greater physical and emotional health.

Polyvagal Practices For Mindfulness And Stress Management

Today's fast-paced world can often leave us overwhelmed, always moving from task to task and keeping our minds filled with an endless list of tasks and responsibilities.

Constant stimulation and exertion can leave us feeling stressed and overburdened, further activating our sympathetic nervous system - the system responsible for our 'fight or flight' response - which in turn activates our sympathetic nervous system, further increasing stress levels and activating it to activate its "fight or flight" response. Unfortunately, pro-longed stress has detrimental consequences both physically and emotionally. However, by leveraging the principles of the Polyvagal Theory, we can cultivate mindfulness and effectively manage stress, navigating our lives with more calmness and clarity.

As improved vagal tone links to lower stress and improved stress management, the methods mentioned before also impacts positively on our stress responses. Let's go over them once more in the context of stress.

Deep Breathing

One of the fundamental practices rooted in Polyvagal Theory for mindfulness and stress management is conscious, deep breathing. Your initial thought might be: How could something so simple have such an enormous effect?

The beauty of this process lies in its simplicity. When we engage in slow, deep and rhythmic breathing, this stimulates the vagus nerve - one of several nerves responsible for switching our body into a restful state of being called parasympathetic nervous system. Even just a few minutes of mindful, deep breathing every day can bring about significant reductions in stress levels.

Yoga And Meditation

Yoga and meditation are other powerful practices that combine physical postures with deep breathing and mindfulness. They offer a holistic approach, enabling us to calm our minds while also engaging our bodies in movement. Mindful-based movements – in contrast to instinctive reactions – actively engage the ventral vagal complex, the center of safety and stability.

In yoga, for instance, the physical postures or 'asanas', combined with conscious, deep breathing, help to cultivate a sense of inner balance and tranquility. Similarly, practices like Tai Chi or Qigong also blend physical movements with mindfulness and controlled breathing, thereby enhancing vagal activity and promoting stress resilience.

Mindfulness meditation, specifically, is a practice which encourages us to remain present and aware without becoming overwhelmed by what's going on around us. Being grounded in the present moment can be an extremely effective means of stress relief.

Studies have demonstrated that mindfulness meditation can increase vagal tone levels, leading to improved emotional regulation and decreased stress levels.

Self-Compassion

As part of our stress management strategies, self-compassion should never be overlooked. By showing kindness towards ourselves with the same respect that we would extend to a close friend, self-compassion can have a powerful positive effect on our mental wellbeing and help create positive shifts in mental state. Self-compassion encourages us to accept and acknowledge our feelings, rather than resist or suppress them. This acceptance is an integral part of mindfulness and is particularly beneficial during stressful times.

Remember, it is not about eliminating stress entirely, which would be an unrealistic expectation. Life will invariably bring challenges and pressures to resolve and act upon. However, by integrating these Polyvagal practices into your routine, you can equip yourself with effective tools to manage stress and navigate life with greater ease and mindfulness. In other words, turn your instinctive reactions into thoughtful actions.

Applying Polyvagal Principles To Sleep And Relaxation

Sleep and relaxation are the next two crucial areas that Poly-vagal practices can positively influence. Sleep is the time when our bodies renew themselves and relax, making it an integral component of overall well-being. Unfortunately, the constant distractions and perpetual busyness of modern life often compromise the quality and quantity of our sleep. It has far-reaching ramifications on our health, affecting everything from mood and cognitive performance to immunity and car-diovascular wellness. It is here that Polyvagal practices can also offer ways to improve our sleep, rest, and relaxation.

To start, let's examine how the Polyvagal Theory relates to sleep. Keep in mind, our nervous system can be divided into two primary branches--sympathetic and parasympathetic.

Simply put, sympathetic nerves control our fight or flight response while parasympathetic nerves handle rest and digest mode.

The Polyvagal Theory proposes that the parasympathetic branch is further divided into two subsystems; of these sub-systems is the vagus nerve or ventral vagal complex (VVC), responsible for social engagement, emotional regulation and more. When the VVC is activated, we are in a state of calm and relaxation, which is optimal for good quality sleep.

So, how can we apply Polyvagal principles to improve sleep? Yet again, we return to an old favorite. Deep, slow breathing stimulates the vagus nerve and helps us enter the 'rest and digest' mode. By including deep breathing exercises into our pre-sleep routine, we can prepare our bodies for an uninterrupted night's rest. To begin, find a comfortable position, close your eyes, and focus on breathing slowly in and slowly out again. Take deep, slow breaths in; hold for several seconds; exhale slowly until breathing out is complete. Repeat this several times, letting go of any tension with each exhale. Try to focus only on your breathing, its rhythm and sensation, while emptying your thoughts as much as possible. No matter the initial difficulty, practice makes perfect!

Furthermore, cultivating a mindful bedtime routine can make a world of difference. This can involve engaging in calming activities such as reading a book, listening to soft music, or practicing gentle yoga. Creating a sleep-friendly environment can also be highly beneficial. This might include ensuring the bedroom is dark, quiet, and cool, using comfortable and supportive bedding, and keeping electronics out of the bedroom.

Another fascinating area to explore is the use of sound to influence the vagus nerve. Chanting and humming are both ways to stimulate the vagus nerve directly due to the connection to the vocal cords and the inner ear. Chanting a simple 'Om' or humming your favorite tune can become part of your relaxation routine. Studies have demonstrated the effectiveness of mindfulness practices for relieving stress, improving mood and aiding in better sleeping patterns.

While we all differ, one size doesn't fit all. It is about experimenting with different strategies and finding what works best for you to build a consistent routine around Sleep is not a luxury but a necessity, and by leveraging Polyvagal principles, we can take steps towards achieving a more restful and restorative sleep experience.

Incorporating Polyvagal Practices Into Your Routine

Let's now consider the practical aspects of integrating Polyvagal practices into your daily routine. Establishing and adhering to a new routine can be challenging. Yet when considering its immense advantages for both physical and mental wellbeing, you will appreciate why taking on such an endeavor is worth your while. Every journey begins with a single step, and integrating Polyvagal practices into your daily life is no exception.

You might ask, "How can I start?" Start small and gradually increase the complexity and duration of your practices. Always remember: **big goals, small steps!** For instance, you can begin by spending just five minutes a day on deep, slow breathing exercises. Gradually, as you become comfortable, you can include other practices like vocal toning or mindfulness exercises into your routine. This gradual approach allows you to gain confidence and foster a sense of achievement, which encourages you to keep going.

A key strategy to maintain consistency is to incorporate Polyvagal practices into activities you already perform daily. Can you practice slow breathing during your commute? Can you perform a short mindfulness exercise before going to bed? By linking Polyvagal practices with existing habits, you are more likely to stick to them.

Always bear in mind that no single approach works for every individual; what works for one may not work for another. So, feel free to experiment and find what practices resonate best with you. It is crucial to make these practices your own, personalizing them to fit your needs, preferences, and lifestyle.

On occasion, you may feel resistant to practicing these mindfulness techniques, and that is perfectly okay – do not judge yourself too harshly when things do not feel quite right! Rather, focus on being kind to yourself instead. Remember, it is about progress, not perfection. If you miss a day, simply resume the next day. Consistency over time is what matters.

Lastly, be patient with yourself. Change may not be apparent immediately, but that does not mean they are not happening. YoAur body and mind are complex systems, and changes at a deep physiological level can take time to manifest as noticeable improvements in your wellbeing.

To conclude, integrating Polyvagal practices into your daily life can yield profound benefits for your physical and mental health. By starting small, linking practices with existing habits, personalizing the practices, and maintaining consistency, you can effectively harness the power of your vagus nerve for your wellbeing. Remember, it is your journey. Be patient, be consistent, and most importantly, enjoy the process. The profound transformation that awaits you is well worth the journey.

In this chapter, we have delved into the practical aspects of Polyvagal Theory. We have explored how to enhance vagal tone, use Polyvagal principles for mindfulness and stress management, apply them to sleep and relaxation, and integrate these practices into your daily routine. By understanding and applying these practices, you are well on your way to unlocking the immense potential of the Polyvagal Theory for your wellbeing.

CONCLUSION

N ow that we have traveled the world of Polyvagal Theory, we appreciate more how its principles and concepts are infused into our overall well-being and everyday lives. The vagus nerves are messengers between the brain and body, sending signals to and from that try to protect their host from danger and increase survival. However, most of these reactions are outside our consciousness and, if unnecessary and exaggerated, become harmful. In other words, if chronic, mental health struggles such as depression, anxiety, and PTSD can develop. In today's world where fear is constantly peddled by politicians, the media, corporations, and activists as a mechanism to control and manipulate people, we cannot easily escape the effects.

That is why the Polyvagal Theory is so important to consider. It provides a mechanism by which knowledge makes people aware that building practices into their daily routines can block and reverse the effects of fear and instability on our bodies and minds.

Do you remember John, the colleague we introduced in the introduction? After seeing him some years later, it was apparent that something had altered him significantly. I inquired further to understand the specifics behind these changes and asked what had occurred since. When answering me, the following explanation came back from him.

Me: Last time we met, I suggested you look into Polyvagal Theory, and I'm curious, did it help you?

John: Absolutely, it has been a game-changer. At first it was difficult for me to grasp what this meant, but once I did so I saw an incredible transformation take place in my life.

Me: That's wonderful, John. Could you please share how it helped you make these changes?

John: Sure. According to this theory, our bodies respond to stress and fear in ways determined by how well our vagus nerve is functioning. When I was struggling before, I often found myself stuck in either fight or flight.

My life became emotionally draining as I constantly prepared to defend myself - making it hard to connect with people around me.

Me: And how did you then apply the Polyvagal Theory to your life?

John: First, I started understanding my triggers - what put me in that fight or flight mode. Then, I worked on ways to help my body feel safe and secure again, such as deep breathing, grounding exercises, yoga, and even simply listening to calming music. Slowly and in stages, I developed a daily routine of the practices that I believed worked for me.

As I started to become more aware of my triggers and reactions to them, I could notice when I was feeling unsafe and act accordingly. Instead of spiraling into anger or isolation, I started to practice self-regulation techniques to calm myself. For instance, just something simple like taking a moment and stepping back when I felt anxiety or anger coming up.

Me: That sounds like a major change. So, did these changes affect your relationships and professional life?

John: Of course, the impact has been remarkable. With a more regulated system, I became less reactive and more proactive. I started having better relationships because I was no longer always on the defense, but rather engaged in understanding others' perspectives. Professionally, I am now able to make decisions without the constant fear of making a mistake. I have regained my confidence, and it has been noted by my team.

Me: That's amazing, John. I'm so thrilled for you!

John: Thank you for guiding my journey in this direction. It has been rewarding indeed. The Polyvagal Theory truly changed my life.

John's testament meant a lot to me in my journey to teach people about the Polyvagal Theory; to allow more people to know and practice these amazing habits. It may take a while, but if you have the patience to build the principles into your daily habits, you can gain similar benefits that John did, and perhaps even more.

www.ingramcontent.com/pod-product-compliance
Lightning Source LLC
Chambersburg PA
CBHW032359280326
41935CB00008B/637